VEGAN GLUTEN-FREE ANTI-INFLAMMATORY COOKBOOK

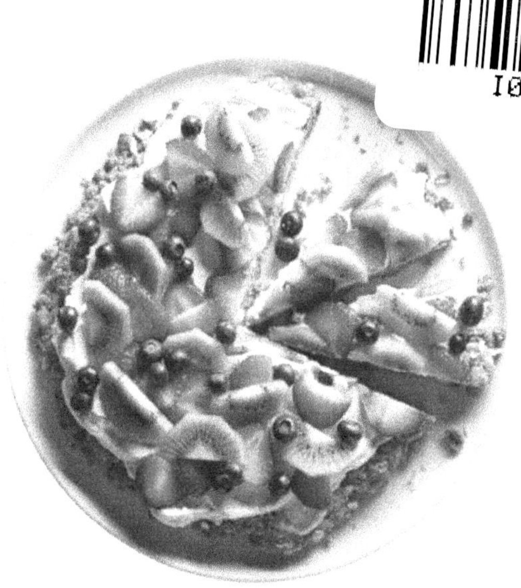

Savoring Easy Delicious Vegan Gluten-Free Meals

Linda Carlucci

Copyright © 2024 by Linda Carlucci

DISCLAIMER

This cookbook is intended to provide general information and recipes.

The recipes provided in this cookbook are not intended to replace or be a substitute for medical advice from a physician.

The reader should consult a healthcare professional for any specific medical advice, diagnosis or treatment.

Any specific dietary advice provided in this cookbook is not intended to replace or be a substitute for medical advice from a physician.

The author is not responsible or liable for any adverse effects experienced by readers of this cookbook as a result of following the recipes or dietary advice provided.

The author makes no representations or warranties of any kind (express or implied) as to the accuracy, completeness, reliability or suitability of the recipes provided in this cookbook.

The author disclaims any and all liability for any damages arising out of the use or misuse of the recipes provided in this cookbook. The reader must also take care to ensure that the recipes provided in this cookbook are prepared and cooked safely.

The recipes provided in this cookbook are for informational purposes only and should not be used as a substitute for professional medical advice, diagnosis or treatment.

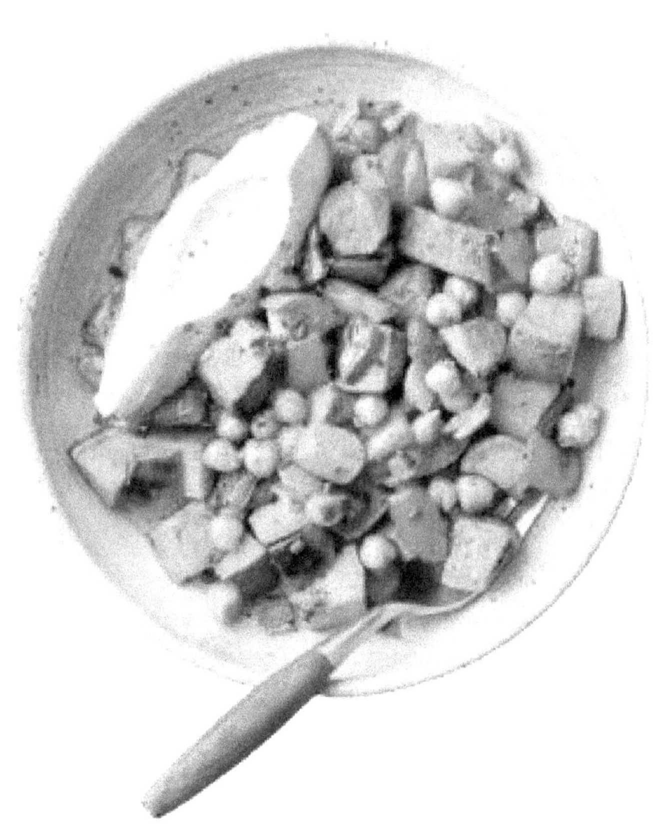

TABLE OF CONTENTS

INTRODUCTION

This book offers a diverse range of delicious recipes designed to support a healthy lifestyle.

It is tailored for you seeking to reduce inflammation in your body while embracing a vegan and gluten-free diet.

Each recipe is carefully crafted to be both flavorful and nutritious, making it easier to maintain a balanced diet.

The cookbook features a variety of breakfast, lunch, dinner, soups and stews and dessert options to suit every palate.

From hearty salads packed with fresh vegetables and protein-rich legumes to comforting soups and stews bursting with flavor, there's something for everyone in this cookbook.

Additionally, the recipes are designed to be simple and easy to follow, making them perfect for both seasoned cooks and beginners alike.

One of the key features of this cookbook is its focus on using whole, plant-based ingredients that are known for their anti-inflammatory properties. Ingredients such as turmeric, ginger, and leafy greens are used generously throughout the recipes to help reduce inflammation and promote overall health. Additionally, the recipes are free from gluten, making them suitable for those with gluten sensitivities or celiac disease.

In addition to delicious recipes, this cookbook also includes valuable information on the benefits of a vegan and gluten-free diet, as well as tips for incorporating more anti-inflammatory foods into your daily meals.

Whether you're looking to improve your health or simply enjoy flavorful, plant-based meals, this cookbook is a must-have for anyone looking to embrace a healthier lifestyle.

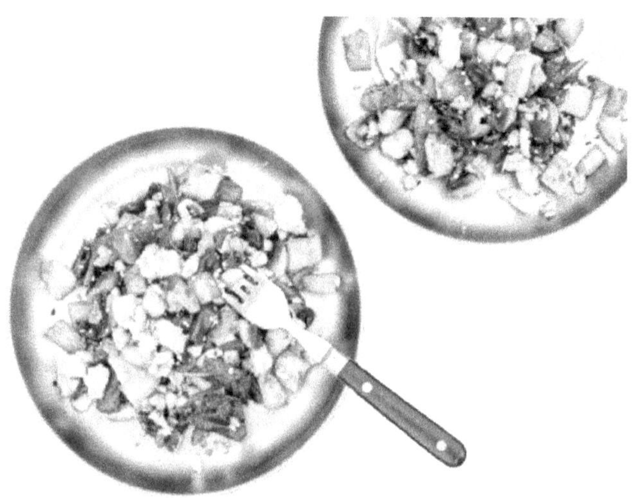

CHAPTER 1

UNDERSTANDING INFLAMMATION AND ITS IMPACT ON THE BODY

Inflammation is a natural process that occurs in the body as a response to injury, infection, or harmful substances.

It is a vital part of the immune system's defense mechanism, helping to protect the body and promote healing.

However, when inflammation becomes chronic, it can have a negative impact on overall health.

Chronic inflammation occurs when the immune system remains activated for an extended period, leading to persistent inflammation throughout the body.

This can be caused by a variety of factors, including poor diet, stress, lack of exercise, and exposure to environmental toxins. Chronic inflammation has been linked to a range of health problems, including heart disease, diabetes, arthritis, and even cancer.

One of the key ways chronic inflammations can impact the body is by damaging tissues and organs over time. This can lead to a variety of health issues, including joint pain, fatigue, and digestive problems.

Chronic inflammation has also been linked to an increased risk of developing certain diseases, such as heart disease and diabetes.

In addition to physical health problems, chronic inflammation can also have a negative impact on mental health.

Studies have shown that chronic inflammation may play a role in the development of depression and other mood disorders.

Fortunately, there are steps that can be taken to reduce inflammation and protect overall health. Eating a healthy diet rich in anti-inflammatory foods, such as fruits, vegetables, whole grains, and healthy fats, can help to reduce inflammation in the body.

Regular exercise, stress management techniques, and avoiding exposure to environmental toxins can also help to reduce inflammation and protect against its negative effects.

HEALTH BENEFITS OF FOLLOWING AN ANTI-INFLAMMATORY DIET

1. **Reduced Risk of Chronic Diseases:** Chronic inflammation is linked to the development of various chronic diseases, including heart disease, diabetes, cancer, and Alzheimer's disease. By reducing inflammation in the body, an anti-inflammatory diet can help lower the risk of developing these conditions.

2. **Improved Joint Health:** Inflammation plays a key role in conditions such as arthritis, which can cause joint pain and stiffness. An anti-inflammatory diet rich in foods like fruits, vegetables, and omega-3 fatty acids can help reduce inflammation in the joints, leading to improved joint health and reduced pain.

3. **Better Digestive Health:** Chronic inflammation in the digestive tract can lead to conditions such as inflammatory bowel disease (IBD) and irritable bowel syndrome (IBS). An anti-inflammatory diet can help soothe inflammation in the gut, leading to

improved digestive health and reduced symptoms of these conditions.

4. **Enhanced Immune Function:** The immune system plays a crucial role in inflammation, and chronic inflammation can weaken the immune system. By following an anti-inflammatory diet, you can help support a healthy immune system and reduce the risk of infections and illnesses.

5. **Weight Management:** Obesity is associated with chronic inflammation, which can contribute to the development of various health conditions. An anti-inflammatory diet can help promote weight loss and weight management, reducing the risk of obesity-related inflammation.

6. **Improved Skin Health:** Inflammation can contribute to skin conditions such as acne, eczema, and psoriasis. An anti-inflammatory diet rich in fruits, vegetables, and healthy fats can help reduce inflammation in the skin, leading to clearer, healthier skin.

FOODS NOT ALLOWED ON AN ANTI-INFLAMMATORY DIET

1. **Processed Foods:** Processed foods are often high in unhealthy fats, sugars, and additives, which can contribute to inflammation in the body. These include fast food, processed meats, and packaged snacks.

2. **Sugary Foods and Beverages:** Foods and beverages high in added sugars can contribute to inflammation and may increase the risk of developing chronic diseases. This includes sugary drinks, candies, and desserts.

3. **Refined Carbohydrates:** Refined carbohydrates, such as white bread, white rice, and pasta, can cause spikes in blood sugar levels, leading to inflammation. It's best to choose whole grains instead.

4. **Trans Fats:** Trans fats are a type of unhealthy fat found in processed and fried foods. They can contribute to inflammation and increase the risk of heart disease. It's important to read food labels and avoid products that contain trans fats.

5. **Vegetable Oils:** Some vegetable oils, such as corn, soybean, and sunflower oils, are high in omega-6 fatty acids, which can promote inflammation when consumed in excess. It's better to choose oils high in omega-3 fatty acids, such as olive oil or flaxseed oil.

6. **Excessive Alcohol:** While moderate alcohol consumption may have some health benefits, excessive alcohol intake can contribute to inflammation and damage to the liver and other organs.

7. **Artificial Additives:** Artificial additives, such as artificial sweeteners, colors, and preservatives, may trigger inflammation in some people. It's best to choose whole, natural foods whenever possible.

EFFECTIVE EXERCISES TO REDUCE INFLAMMATION

1. **Cardiovascular Exercise:** Aerobic exercises such as walking, jogging, cycling, and swimming can help reduce inflammation by improving circulation and promoting the release of anti-inflammatory compounds in the body.

CHAPTER 2

14-DAY MEAL PLAN

DAY 1

Breakfast: Quinoa Breakfast Bowl with Mixed Berries

Lunch: Roasted Vegetable Quinoa Salad

Dinner: Black Bean and Quinoa Stuffed Peppers with Chipotle Sauce

DAY 2

Breakfast: Turmeric Tofu Scramble

Lunch: Vegan Lentil Soup with Turmeric and Kale

Dinner: Curried Chickpea Salad Wraps with Spinach and Avocado

DAY 3

Breakfast: Chia Seed Pudding with Mango and Coconut

Lunch: Zucchini Noodles with Avocado Pesto

Dinner: Portobello Mushroom Burgers with Onions and Guacamole

DAY 4

Breakfast: Sweet Potato Hash with Chickpeas

Lunch: Chickpea Salad Sandwiches on Gluten-Free Bread

Dinner: Rainbow Veggie Spring Rolls with Peanut Dipping Sauce

DAY 5

Breakfast: Breakfast Hash with Chickpeas

Lunch: Spicy Sweet Potato and Black Bean Tacos

Dinner: Moroccan Chickpea Tagine with Apricots and Almonds

DAY 6

Breakfast: Vegan Gluten-Free Pancakes

Lunch: Mediterranean Stuffed Bell Peppers with Quinoa and Olives

Dinner: Stuffed Bell Peppers with Quinoa, Black Beans, and Roasted Corn

DAY 7

Breakfast: Avocado Toast with Hemp Seeds

Lunch: Thai Coconut Curry Soup with Tofu and Vegetable

Dinner: Portobello Mushroom Steaks with Chimichurri Sauce

DAY 8

Breakfast: Buckwheat Porridge with Almond Butter

Lunch: Cauliflower Rice Sushi Rolls with Mango and Cucumber

Dinner: Thai Green Curry with Tofu and Vegetables

DAY 9

Breakfast: Coconut Yogurt Parfait with Granola

Lunch: Butternut Squash and Kale Salad with Maple-Dijon Dressing

Dinner: Eggplant Rollatini with Vegan Ricotta and Marinara Sauce

DAY 10

Breakfast: Green Smoothie Bowl with Kale and Flaxseeds

Lunch: Vegan Gluten-Free Pizza with Spinach and Sun-Dried Tomatoes

Dinner: Teriyaki Tempeh Stir-Fry with Broccoli and Bell Peppers

DAY 11

Breakfast: Quinoa Breakfast Bowl with Mixed Berries

Lunch: Roasted Vegetable Quinoa Salad

Dinner: Black Bean and Quinoa Stuffed Peppers with Chipotle Sauce

DAY 12

Breakfast: Turmeric Tofu Scramble

Lunch: Vegan Lentil Soup with Turmeric and Kale

Dinner: Curried Chickpea Salad Wraps with Spinach and Avocado

DAY 13

Breakfast: Chia Seed Pudding with Mango and Coconut

Lunch: Zucchini Noodles with Avocado Pesto

Dinner: Portobello Mushroom Burgers with Onions and Guacamole

Breakfast: Sweet Potato Hash with Chickpeas

Lunch: Chickpea Salad Sandwiches on Gluten-Free Bread

Dinner: Rainbow Veggie Spring Rolls with Peanut Dipping Sauce

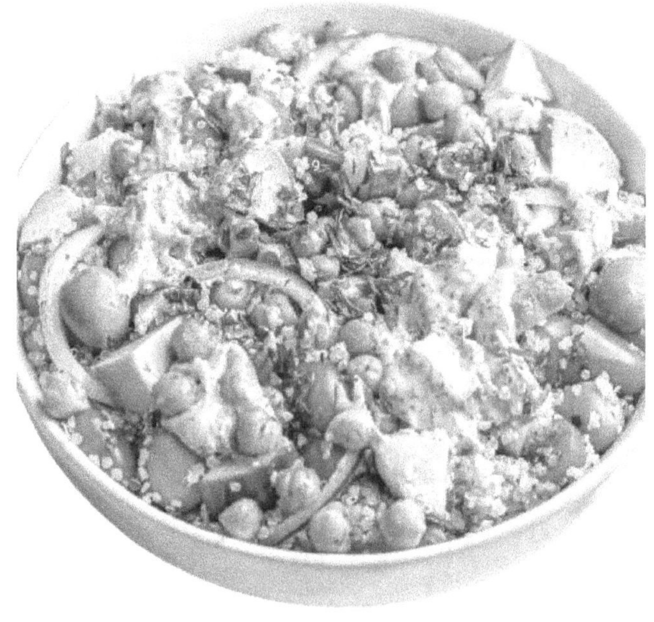

CHAPTER 3

NUTRITIOUS RECIPES FOR A VEGAN CLUTEN-FREE ANTI-INFLAMMATORY DIET

BREAKFAST

Quinoa Breakfast Bowl with Mixed Berries

Preparation Time: 5 minutes

Serves: 4

Calories: 300 **Carbs:** 45g **Protein:** 9g **Fat:** 9g **Fiber:** 7g **Sodium:** 120mg

Ingredients:

1 cup quinoa

2 cups almond milk

1 tablespoon maple syrup

1 teaspoon vanilla extract

1 cup mixed berries (such as strawberries, blueberries, raspberries)

1 tablespoon chia seeds

1 tablespoon hemp seeds

1 tablespoon chopped walnuts

Method of Preparation:

1. Rinse the quinoa under cold water.
2. In a medium saucepan, combine the quinoa, almond milk, maple syrup, and vanilla extract.
3. Bring to a boil, then reduce the heat to low and simmer for 15-20 minutes, or until the quinoa is cooked and the liquid is absorbed.
4. Divide the quinoa into bowls and top with mixed berries, chia seeds, hemp seeds, and chopped walnuts.
5. Serve hot.

Turmeric Tofu Scramble

Preparation Time: 10 minutes

Serves: 4

Calories: 180 **Carbs:** 8g **Protein:** 12g **Fat:** 12g **Fiber:** 3g **Sodium:** 80mg

Ingredients:

1 block (14 oz) firm tofu, drained and crumbled

1 tablespoon olive oil

1 onion, diced

1 bell pepper, diced

2 teaspoons turmeric powder

1 teaspoon garlic powder

1 teaspoon cumin powder

A pinch of salt and pepper

Fresh parsley, for garnish

Method of Preparation:

1. Heat the olive oil in a large skillet over medium heat.
2. Add the onion and bell pepper, and sauté until softened, about 5 minutes.
3. Add the crumbled tofu, turmeric powder, garlic powder, cumin powder, salt, and pepper.

4. Cook, stirring occasionally, for another 5-7 minutes, or until the tofu is heated through and well coated with the spices.

5. Garnish with fresh parsley before serving.

Chia Seed Pudding with Mango and Coconut

Preparation Time: 5 minutes (+ refrigeration time)

Serves: 2

Calories: 220 **Carbs:** 26g **Protein:** 5g **Fat:** 12g **Fiber:** 10g **Sodium:** 100mg

Ingredients:

1/4 cup chia seeds

1 cup almond milk

1 tablespoon maple syrup

1/2 teaspoon vanilla extract

1/2 cup diced mango

2 tablespoons shredded coconut

Method of Preparation:

1. In a bowl, combine the chia seeds, almond milk, maple syrup, and vanilla extract.
2. Stir well to combine, then cover and refrigerate for at least 4 hours, or overnight, until the mixture thickens and becomes pudding-like.
3. Divide the pudding into serving bowls and top with diced mango and shredded coconut.
4. Serve chilled.

Sweet Potato Hash with Chickpeas

Preparation Time: 10 minutes

Serves: 4

Calories: 320 **Carbs:** 50g **Protein:** 9g **Fat:** 10g **Fiber:** 10g **Sodium:** 330mg

Ingredients:

2 large sweet potatoes, peeled and diced

1 can (15 oz) chickpeas, drained and rinsed

1 onion, diced

1 bell pepper, diced

2 tablespoons olive oil

1 teaspoon smoked paprika

1/2 teaspoon cumin

A pinch of salt and pepper

Fresh parsley, for garnish

Method of Preparation:

1. Heat olive oil in a large skillet over medium heat.
2. Add onion and bell pepper, and sauté until softened, about 5 minutes.
3. Add sweet potatoes, chickpeas, smoked paprika, cumin, salt, and pepper.
4. Cook, stirring occasionally, for about 15-20 minutes, or until sweet potatoes are tender and chickpeas are slightly crispy.
5. Garnish with fresh parsley before serving.

Breakfast Hash with Chickpeas

Preparation Time: 10 minutes

Serves: 4

Calories: 280 **Carbs:** 45g **Protein:** 9g **Fat:** 8g **Fiber:** 8g
Sodium: 310mg

Ingredients:

2 cups diced potatoes

1 can (15 oz) chickpeas, drained and rinsed

1 onion, diced

1 bell pepper, diced

2 tablespoons olive oil

1 teaspoon garlic powder

1 teaspoon paprika

A pinch of salt and pepper

Fresh cilantro, for garnish

Method of Preparation:

1. Heat olive oil in a large skillet over medium heat.
2. Add onion and bell pepper, and sauté until softened, about 5 minutes.
3. Add potatoes, chickpeas, garlic powder, paprika, salt, and pepper.
4. Cook, stirring occasionally, for about 15-20 minutes, or until potatoes are tender and slightly crispy.
5. Garnish with fresh cilantro before serving.

Vegan Gluten-Free Pancakes

Preparation Time: 10 minutes

Serves: 4 (3 pancakes per serving)

Calories: 280 **Carbs:** 45g **Protein:** 5g **Fat:** 8g **Fiber:** 6g **Sodium:** 320mg

Ingredients:

1 cup gluten-free flour

1 tablespoon baking powder

1/4 teaspoon salt

1 tablespoon maple syrup

1 cup almond milk

1 tablespoon apple cider vinegar

1 tablespoon coconut oil, melted

Fresh berries, for topping

Maple syrup, for drizzling

Method of Preparation:

1. In a bowl, whisk together gluten-free flour, baking powder, and salt.
2. In a separate bowl, mix maple syrup, almond milk, apple cider vinegar, and melted coconut oil.
3. Pour wet ingredients into dry ingredients and stir until just combined.
4. Heat a non-stick skillet over medium heat.
5. Pour 1/4 cup of batter onto the skillet and cook until bubbles form on the surface.
6. Flip and cook for another 1-2 minutes, or until cooked through.
7. Repeat with remaining batter.

8. Serve pancakes topped with fresh berries and maple syrup.

Avocado Toast with Hemp Seeds

Preparation Time: 5 minutes

Serves: 1

Calories: 320 **Carbs:** 25g **Protein:** 9g **Fat:** 22g **Fiber:** 13g **Sodium:** 250mg

Ingredients:

2 slices gluten-free bread

1 ripe avocado

2 tablespoons hemp seeds

A pinch of salt and pepper

Red pepper flakes, for garnish (optional)

Method of Preparation:

1. Toast the gluten-free bread slices until golden brown.
2. Mash the ripe avocado in a bowl and season with salt and pepper.

3. Spread the mashed avocado evenly on the toasted bread slices.

4. Sprinkle hemp seeds on top of the avocado mash.

5. Garnish with red pepper flakes, if desired.

Buckwheat Porridge with Almond Butter

Preparation Time: 5 minutes

Serves: 2

Calories: 280 **Carbs:** 45g **Protein:** 9g **Fat:** 8g **Fiber:** 6g **Sodium:** 150mg

Ingredients:

1/2 cup buckwheat groats

1 cup almond milk

1 tablespoon almond butter

1 tablespoon maple syrup

1/2 teaspoon cinnamon

Fresh berries, for topping

Method of Preparation:

1. Rinse the buckwheat groats under cold water.
2. In a saucepan, combine the rinsed buckwheat groats and almond milk.
3. Bring to a boil, then reduce the heat to low and simmer for 10-15 minutes, or until the buckwheat is tender.
4. Stir in almond butter, maple syrup, and cinnamon.
5. Serve the porridge topped with fresh berries.

Coconut Yogurt Parfait with Granola

Preparation Time: 5 minutes

Serves: 1

Calories: 350 **Carbs:** 45g **Protein:** 6g **Fat:** 15g **Fiber:** 8g **Sodium:** 50mg

Ingredients:

1 cup coconut yogurt

1/2 cup gluten-free granola

1/2 cup mixed berries

1 tablespoon chia seeds

Method of Preparation:

1. In a glass or bowl, layer coconut yogurt, gluten-free granola, mixed berries, and chia seeds.
2. Repeat the layers until all ingredients are used up.
3. Serve immediately.

Green Smoothie Bowl with Kale and Flaxseeds

Preparation Time: 5 minutes

Serves: 1

Calories: 300 **Carbs:** 40g **Protein:** 8g **Fat:** 15g **Fiber:** 10g **Sodium:** 100mg

Ingredients:

1 cup kale leaves, stems removed

1/2 banana

1/2 cup almond milk

1 tablespoon flaxseeds

1/2 cup frozen mixed berries

1 tablespoon almond butter

Fresh fruit, nuts, and seeds, for topping

Method of Preparation:

1. In a blender, combine kale leaves, banana, almond milk, flaxseeds, frozen mixed berries, and almond butter.
2. Blend until smooth and creamy.
3. Pour the smoothie into a bowl and top with fresh fruit, nuts, and seeds.
4. Serve immediately.

LUNCH

Roasted Vegetable Quinoa Salad

Preparation Time: 15 minutes

Serves: 4

Calories: 320 **Carbs:** 45g **Protein:** 8g **Fat:** 12g **Fiber:** 7g **Sodium:** 100mg

Ingredients:

1 cup quinoa

2 cups vegetable broth

1 red bell pepper, chopped

1 yellow bell pepper, chopped

1 zucchini, chopped

1 yellow squash, chopped

1 red onion, chopped

2 tablespoons olive oil

1 teaspoon smoked paprika

A pinch of salt and pepper

1/4 cup fresh parsley, chopped

Juice of 1 lemon

Method of Preparation:

1. Preheat the oven to 400°F (200°C).
2. In a large bowl, toss the chopped vegetables with olive oil, smoked paprika, salt, and pepper.

3. Spread the vegetables in a single layer on a baking sheet lined with parchment paper.

4. Roast in the preheated oven for 25-30 minutes, or until vegetables are tender and slightly caramelized.

5. In a medium saucepan, combine quinoa and vegetable broth.

6. Bring to a boil, then reduce heat and simmer for 15-20 minutes, or until quinoa is cooked and liquid is absorbed.

7. In a large bowl, combine cooked quinoa, roasted vegetables, chopped parsley, and lemon juice.

8. Toss to combine.

9. Serve warm or at room temperature.

Vegan Lentil Soup with Turmeric and Kale

Preparation Time: 10 minutes

Serves: 6

Calories: 250 **Carbs:** 40g **Protein:** 15g **Fat:** 5g **Fiber:** 10g **Sodium:** 100mg

Ingredients:

1 tablespoon olive oil

1 onion, chopped

2 carrots, chopped

2 celery stalks, chopped

2 garlic cloves, minced

1 teaspoon turmeric powder

1 cup green or brown lentils, rinsed and drained

6 cups vegetable broth

1 can (14 oz) diced tomatoes

2 cups chopped kale

A pinch of salt and pepper

Fresh parsley, for garnish

Method of Preparation:

1. In a large pot, heat olive oil over medium heat.
2. Add onion, carrots, celery, and garlic.

3. Sauté until vegetables are softened, about 5-7 minutes.

4. Stir in turmeric powder and cook for another minute.

5. Add lentils, vegetable broth, and diced tomatoes.

6. Bring to a boil, then reduce heat and simmer for 20-25 minutes, or until lentils are tender.

7. Stir in chopped kale and cook for another 5 minutes, or until kale is wilted.

8. Season with A pinch of salt and pepper.

9. Serve hot, garnished with fresh parsley.

Zucchini Noodles with Avocado Pesto

Preparation Time: 10 minutes

Serves: 2

Calories: 320 **Carbs:** 20g **Protein:** 8g **Fat:** 25g **Fiber:** 10g **Sodium:** 150mg

Ingredients:

2 large zucchinis, spiralized into noodles

1 ripe avocado

1/4 cup fresh basil leaves

1/4 cup fresh parsley leaves

1/4 cup walnuts

2 tablespoons lemon juice

1 garlic clove

2 tablespoons olive oil

A pinch of salt and pepper

Cherry tomatoes, halved, for garnish

Method of Preparation:

1. In a blender or food processor, combine avocado, basil, parsley, walnuts, lemon juice, garlic, olive oil, salt, and pepper. Blend until smooth and creamy.

2. In a large bowl, toss the zucchini noodles with the avocado pesto until well coated.

3. Serve the zucchini noodles topped with cherry tomatoes.

Chickpea Salad Sandwiches on Gluten-Free Bread

Preparation Time: 10 minutes

Serves: 4

Calories: 150 **Carbs:** 20g **Protein:** 5g **Fat:** 6g **Fiber:** 6g **Sodium:** 100mg

Ingredients:

1 can (15 oz) chickpeas, drained and rinsed

1/4 cup vegan mayonnaise

1 tablespoon Dijon mustard

1 celery stalk, finely chopped

1/4 cup red onion, finely chopped

1/4 cup fresh parsley, chopped

A pinch of salt and pepper

Gluten-free bread slices

Lettuce leaves, for serving

Tomato slices, for serving

Method of Preparation:

1. In a large bowl, mash the chickpeas with a fork or potato masher.
2. Add vegan mayonnaise, Dijon mustard, celery, red onion, parsley, salt, and pepper.
3. Stir until well combined.
4. Toast the gluten-free bread slices, if desired.
5. Spread the chickpea salad on one slice of bread.
6. Top with lettuce leaves and tomato slices.
7. Place another slice of bread on top to make a sandwich.
8. Serve immediately.

Spicy Sweet Potato and Black Bean Tacos

Preparation Time: 10 minutes

Serves: 4

Calories: 300 **Carbs:** 50g **Protein:** 8g **Fat:** 8g **Fiber:** 10g **Sodium:** 50mg

Ingredients:

2 medium sweet potatoes, peeled and diced

1 tablespoon olive oil

1 teaspoon chili powder

1/2 teaspoon cumin

1/2 teaspoon paprika

A pinch of salt and pepper

1 can (15 oz) black beans, drained and rinsed

8 gluten-free corn tortillas

Salsa, avocado, and cilantro, for serving

Method of Preparation:

1. Preheat the oven to 400°F (200°C).
2. In a large bowl, toss the sweet potatoes with olive oil, chili powder, cumin, paprika, salt, and pepper.
3. Spread the sweet potatoes in a single layer on a baking sheet lined with parchment paper.

4. Roast in the preheated oven for 20-25 minutes, or until sweet potatoes are tender and slightly caramelized.

5. In a small saucepan, heat the black beans until warmed through.

6. Heat the corn tortillas in a dry skillet over medium heat for about 30 seconds per side.

7. Assemble the tacos by filling each tortilla with roasted sweet potatoes, black beans, salsa, avocado, and cilantro.

8. Serve immediately.

Mediterranean Stuffed Bell Peppers with Quinoa and Olives

Preparation Time: 15 minutes

Serves: 4

Calories: 300 **Carbs:** 45g **Protein:** 10g **Fat:** 10g **Fiber:** 12g **Sodium:** 100mg

Ingredients:

4 large bell peppers, halved and seeds removed

1 cup cooked quinoa

1 can (15 oz) chickpeas, drained and rinsed

1/2 cup diced cucumber

1/4 cup chopped Kalamata olives

1/4 cup chopped fresh parsley

2 tablespoons lemon juice

2 tablespoons olive oil

A pinch of salt and pepper

Method of Preparation:

1. Preheat the oven to 375°F (190°C).
2. Place the bell pepper halves on a baking sheet lined with parchment paper.
3. In a large bowl, combine cooked quinoa, chickpeas, cucumber, olives, parsley, lemon juice, olive oil, salt, and pepper.
4. Spoon the quinoa mixture into the bell pepper halves.
5. Cover the baking sheet with foil and bake in the preheated oven for 25-30 minutes, or until the bell peppers are tender.

6. Serve hot.

Thai Coconut Curry Soup with Tofu and Vegetables

Preparation Time: 15 minutes

Serves: 4

Calories: 350 **Carbs:** 20g **Protein:** 15g **Fat:** 25g **Fiber:** 5g **Sodium:** 100mg

Ingredients:

1 tablespoon coconut oil

1 onion, chopped

2 garlic cloves, minced

1 tablespoon grated ginger

2 tablespoons Thai red curry paste

1 can (14 oz) coconut milk

4 cups vegetable broth

1 block (14 oz) firm tofu, diced

2 cups mixed vegetables (such as bell peppers, broccoli, and snap peas)

1 tablespoon soy sauce

1 tablespoon maple syrup

Juice of 1 lime

Fresh cilantro, for garnish

Cooked rice or noodles, for serving

Method of Preparation:

1. In a large pot, heat coconut oil over medium heat.
2. Add onion, garlic, and ginger.
3. Sauté until onion is translucent, about 5 minutes.
4. Stir in Thai red curry paste and cook for another minute.
5. Add coconut milk and vegetable broth. Bring to a simmer.
6. Add tofu, mixed vegetables, soy sauce, and maple syrup.
7. Cook for 10-15 minutes, or until vegetables are tender.
8. Stir in lime juice.

9. Serve hot, garnished with fresh cilantro, over cooked rice or noodles.

Cauliflower Rice Sushi Rolls with Mango and Cucumber

Preparation Time: 20 minutes

Serves: 4

Calories: 100 **Carbs:** 20g **Protein:** 3g **Fat:** 1g **Fiber:** 5g **Sodium:** 60mg

Ingredients:

1 head cauliflower, riced

1 mango, thinly sliced

1 cucumber, julienned

4 nori sheets

Soy sauce, for serving

Pickled ginger, for serving

Wasabi, for serving

Method of Preparation:

1. Spread a thin layer of cauliflower rice on a nori sheet.
2. Top with mango slices and cucumber sticks.
3. Roll up the nori sheet tightly, using a bamboo sushi mat if available.
4. Repeat with the remaining ingredients.
5. Slice the rolls into bite-sized pieces.
6. Serve with soy sauce, pickled ginger, and wasabi.

Butternut Squash and Kale Salad with Maple-Dijon Dressing

Preparation Time: 20 minutes

Serves: 4

Calories: 250 **Carbs:** 30g **Protein:** 5g **Fat:** 15g **Fiber:** 5g **Sodium:** 80mg

Ingredients:

1 small butternut squash, peeled, seeded, and cubed

1 tablespoon olive oil

A pinch of salt and pepper

4 cups chopped kale

1/4 cup dried cranberries

1/4 cup chopped walnuts

1/4 cup crumbled vegan feta cheese (optional)

Maple-Dijon Dressing:

2 tablespoons olive oil

1 tablespoon apple cider vinegar

1 tablespoon maple syrup

1 teaspoon Dijon mustard

A pinch of salt and pepper

Method of Preparation:

1. Preheat the oven to 400°F (200°C).
2. Toss butternut squash cubes with olive oil, salt, and pepper.
3. Spread the squash on a baking sheet lined with parchment paper.
4. Roast in the preheated oven for 25-30 minutes, or until tender and caramelized.

5. In a large bowl, massage kale with a little olive oil to soften.

6. Add roasted butternut squash, dried cranberries, chopped walnuts, and vegan feta cheese.

7. In a small bowl, whisk together olive oil, apple cider vinegar, maple syrup, Dijon mustard, salt, and pepper to make the dressing.

8. Drizzle the dressing over the salad and toss to combine.

9. Serve at room temperature.

Vegan Gluten-Free Pizza with Spinach and Sun-Dried Tomatoes

Preparation Time: 15 minutes

Serves: 4

Calories: 300 **Carbs:** 40g **Protein:** 5g **Fat:** 15g **Fiber:** 5g **Sodium:** 100mg

Ingredients:

1 gluten-free pizza crust

1/2 cup tomato sauce

1 cup fresh spinach

1/4 cup sun-dried tomatoes, chopped

1/4 cup sliced black olives

1/4 cup sliced red onion

1/2 cup vegan mozzarella cheese, shredded

Fresh basil, for garnish

Red pepper flakes, for garnish

Method of Preparation:

1. Preheat the oven according to the pizza crust instructions.
2. Spread tomato sauce over the pizza crust.
3. Top with spinach, sun-dried tomatoes, black olives, red onion, and vegan mozzarella cheese.
4. Bake in the preheated oven for 10-15 minutes, or until the crust is golden and the cheese is melted.
5. Garnish with fresh basil and red pepper flakes before serving.

DINNER

Black Bean and Quinoa Stuffed Peppers with Chipotle Sauce

Preparation Time: 20 minutes

Serves: 4

Calories: 300 **Carbs:** 55g **Protein:** 12g **Fat:** 3g **Fiber:** 12g **Sodium:** 100mg

Ingredients:

4 large bell peppers, halved and seeds removed

1 cup cooked quinoa

1 can (15 oz) black beans, drained and rinsed

1 cup corn kernels

1/2 cup diced tomatoes

1/2 cup diced red onion

1/2 cup chopped cilantro

1 teaspoon cumin

1 teaspoon chili powder

A pinch of salt and pepper

1/2 cup chipotle sauce (store-bought or homemade)

Method of Preparation:

1. Preheat the oven to 375°F (190°C).
2. In a large bowl, combine cooked quinoa, black beans, corn, tomatoes, red onion, cilantro, cumin, chili powder, salt, and pepper.
3. Spoon the quinoa mixture into the bell pepper halves.
4. Place the stuffed peppers in a baking dish and cover with foil.
5. Bake in the preheated oven for 25-30 minutes, or until the peppers are tender.
6. Serve hot, drizzled with chipotle sauce.

Curried Chickpea Salad Wraps with Spinach and Avocado

Preparation Time: 15 minutes

Serves: 4

Calories: 400 **Carbs:** 45g **Protein:** 10g **Fat:** 20g **Fiber:** 10g **Sodium:** 100mg

Ingredients:

1 can (15 oz) chickpeas, drained and rinsed

1/2 cup vegan mayonnaise

1 tablespoon curry powder

1/2 cup diced red onion

1/2 cup diced celery

1/4 cup chopped fresh cilantro

A pinch of salt and pepper

4 large spinach wraps

1 avocado, sliced

Method of Preparation:

1. In a large bowl, mash the chickpeas with a fork.
2. Add vegan mayonnaise, curry powder, red onion, celery, cilantro, salt, and pepper.
3. Stir until well combined.

4. Place a scoop of the chickpea salad onto a spinach wrap.

5. Top with avocado slices.

6. Roll up the wrap tightly, tucking in the sides as you go.

7. Slice the wrap in half and serve.

Portobello Mushroom Burgers with Onions and Guacamole

Preparation Time: 15 minutes

Serves: 4

Calories: 350 **Carbs:** 40g **Protein:** 8g **Fat:** 18g **Fiber:** 10g **Sodium:** 100mg

Ingredients:

4 large portobello mushroom caps

2 tablespoons olive oil

1 teaspoon smoked paprika

A pinch of salt and pepper

1 red onion, sliced

4 gluten-free burger buns

Guacamole, for topping

Method of Preparation:

1. Preheat the grill or a grill pan over medium-high heat.
2. In a small bowl, whisk together olive oil, smoked paprika, salt, and pepper.
3. Brush the mushroom caps with the olive oil mixture.
4. Grill the mushroom caps for 4-5 minutes per side, or until tender.
5. In the meantime, grill the sliced red onion until softened and slightly charred.
6. Toast the burger buns on the grill, if desired.
7. Assemble the burgers by placing a grilled mushroom cap on the bottom half of each bun.
8. Top with grilled red onion and guacamole.
9. Place the top half of the bun on top.
10. Serve immediately.

Rainbow Veggie Spring Rolls with Peanut Dipping Sauce

Preparation Time: 20 minutes

Serves: 4

Calories: 250 **Carbs:** 35g **Protein:** 7g **Fat:** 9g **Fiber:** 6g **Sodium:** 100mg

Ingredients:

8 rice paper wrappers

2 cups mixed veggies (such as bell peppers, carrots, cucumber, and avocado), julienned

1/2 cup fresh herbs (such as mint, cilantro, and basil), chopped

1/2 cup cooked rice noodles

Peanut dipping sauce (see below)

Peanut Dipping Sauce:

1/4 cup peanut butter

2 tablespoons soy sauce

1 tablespoon maple syrup

1 tablespoon lime juice

1 garlic clove, minced

Water, as needed

Method of Preparation:

1. Prepare the peanut dipping sauce by whisking together all the ingredients in a bowl.
2. Add water as needed to reach desired consistency. Set aside.
3. Fill a large bowl with warm water. Dip one rice paper wrapper into the water for a few seconds until it softens.
4. Place the softened wrapper on a clean surface. Arrange a small handful of mixed veggies, herbs, and rice noodles in the center of the wrapper.
5. Fold the sides of the wrapper over the filling, then roll up tightly.
6. Repeat with the remaining wrappers and filling ingredients.
7. Serve the spring rolls with the peanut dipping sauce.

Moroccan Chickpea Tagine with Apricots and Almonds

Preparation Time: 15 minutes

Serves: 4

Calories: 300 **Carbs:** 45g **Protein:** 10g **Fat:** 10g **Fiber:** 12g **Sodium:** 100mg

Ingredients:

1 tablespoon olive oil

1 onion, chopped

2 garlic cloves, minced

1 tablespoon grated ginger

1 tablespoon Moroccan spice blend (or a mix of cumin, coriander, cinnamon, and paprika)

1 can (15 oz) chickpeas, drained and rinsed

1 can (14 oz) diced tomatoes

1/2 cup dried apricots, chopped

1/4 cup slivered almonds

A pinch of salt and pepper

Fresh cilantro, for garnish

Cooked couscous or quinoa, for serving

Method of Preparation:

1. Heat olive oil in a large pot over medium heat.
2. Add onion, garlic, and ginger.
3. Sauté until onion is translucent, about 5 minutes.
4. Stir in the Moroccan spice blend and cook for another minute.
5. Add chickpeas, diced tomatoes (with juice), and dried apricots.
6. Bring to a simmer.
7. Cover and simmer for 15-20 minutes, stirring occasionally.
8. Stir in slivered almonds and season with salt and pepper.
9. Serve the tagine over cooked couscous or quinoa, garnished with fresh cilantro.

Stuffed Bell Peppers with Quinoa, Black Beans, and Roasted Corn

Preparation Time: 20 minutes

Serves: 4

Calories: 300 **Carbs:** 55g **Protein:** 12g **Fat:** 3g **Fiber:** 12g **Sodium:** 100mg

Ingredients:

4 large bell peppers, halved and seeds removed

1 cup cooked quinoa

1 can (15 oz) black beans, drained and rinsed

1 cup roasted corn kernels

1/2 cup diced tomatoes

1/2 cup diced red onion

1/2 cup chopped cilantro

1 teaspoon cumin

1 teaspoon chili powder

A pinch of salt and pepper

Fresh lime wedges, for serving

Method of Preparation:

1. Preheat the oven to 375°F (190°C).
2. In a large bowl, combine cooked quinoa, black beans, roasted corn, tomatoes, red onion, cilantro, cumin, chili powder, salt, and pepper.
3. Spoon the quinoa mixture into the bell pepper halves.
4. Place the stuffed peppers in a baking dish and cover with foil.
5. Bake in the preheated oven for 25-30 minutes, or until the peppers are tender.
6. Serve hot, with fresh lime wedges.

Portobello Mushroom Steaks with Chimichurri Sauce

Preparation Time: 15 minutes

Serves: 4

Calories: 150 **Carbs:** 10g **Protein:** 5g **Fat:** 10g **Fiber:** 3g **Sodium:** 100mg

Ingredients:

4 large portobello mushroom caps

2 tablespoons olive oil

2 garlic cloves, minced

1/4 cup chopped fresh parsley

2 tablespoons chopped fresh cilantro

2 tablespoons red wine vinegar

1/4 teaspoon red pepper flakes

A pinch of salt and pepper

Chimichurri Sauce:

1/2 cup chopped fresh parsley

1/4 cup chopped fresh cilantro

2 garlic cloves, minced

2 tablespoons red wine vinegar

1/4 cup olive oil

A pinch of salt and pepper

Method of Preparation:

1. Preheat the grill or a grill pan over medium-high heat.

2. Brush the portobello mushroom caps with olive oil and minced garlic.

3. Grill the mushroom caps for 4-5 minutes per side, or until tender.

4. In a small bowl, combine chopped parsley, chopped cilantro, red wine vinegar, red pepper flakes, salt, and pepper. Set aside.

5. For the chimichurri sauce, combine chopped parsley, chopped cilantro, minced garlic, red wine vinegar, olive oil, salt, and pepper in a blender or food processor. Blend until smooth.

6. Serve the grilled portobello mushroom steaks topped with chimichurri sauce.

Thai Green Curry with Tofu and Vegetables

Preparation Time: 20 minutes

Serves: 4

Calories: 300 **Carbs:** 15g **Protein:** 15g **Fat:** 20g **Fiber:** 5g **Sodium:** 100mg

Ingredients:

1 tablespoon coconut oil

1 onion, chopped

2 garlic cloves, minced

1 tablespoon grated ginger

2 tablespoons Thai green curry paste

1 can (14 oz) coconut milk

2 cups vegetable broth

1 block (14 oz) firm tofu, diced

2 cups mixed vegetables (such as bell peppers, broccoli, and snow peas)

1 tablespoon soy sauce

1 tablespoon maple syrup

Juice of 1 lime

Fresh cilantro, for garnish

Cooked rice, for serving

Method of Preparation:

1. In a large pot, heat coconut oil over medium heat.
2. Add onion, garlic, and ginger.
3. Sauté until onion is translucent, about 5 minutes.
4. Stir in Thai green curry paste and cook for another minute.
5. Add coconut milk and vegetable broth.
6. Bring to a simmer.
7. Add tofu, mixed vegetables, soy sauce, and maple syrup.
8. Cook for 10-15 minutes, or until vegetables are tender.
9. Stir in lime juice.
10. Serve hot, garnished with fresh cilantro, over cooked rice.

Eggplant Rollatini with Vegan Ricotta and Marinara Sauce

Preparation Time: 20 minutes

Serves: 4

Calories: 250 **Carbs:** 20g **Protein:** 10g **Fat:** 15g **Fiber:** 8g **Sodium:** 100mg

Ingredients:

1 large eggplant, thinly sliced lengthwise

2 cups vegan ricotta cheese

1/4 cup chopped fresh basil

1/4 cup chopped fresh parsley

A pinch of salt and pepper

2 cups marinara sauce

Method of Preparation:

1. Preheat the oven to 375°F (190°C).
2. Lay the eggplant slices on a baking sheet lined with parchment paper.
3. Bake for 15-20 minutes, or until softened.
4. In a bowl, combine vegan ricotta cheese, chopped basil, chopped parsley, salt, and pepper.
5. Place a spoonful of the ricotta mixture on each eggplant slice and roll up.

6. Spread a thin layer of marinara sauce on the bottom of a baking dish.

7. Place the eggplant rollatini in the dish.

8. Pour the remaining marinara sauce over the rollatini.

9. Bake in the preheated oven for 20-25 minutes, or until heated through.

10. Serve hot.

Teriyaki Tempeh Stir-Fry with Broccoli and Bell Peppers

Preparation Time: 15 minutes

Serves: 4

Calories: 300 **Carbs:** 15g **Protein:** 15g **Fat:** 20g **Fiber:** 5g **Sodium:** 100mg

Ingredients:

1 tablespoon sesame oil

1 block (8 oz) tempeh, cubed

2 cups broccoli florets

1 bell pepper, sliced

1/4 cup teriyaki sauce

Cooked brown rice, for serving

Sesame seeds, for garnish

Method of Preparation:

1. In a large skillet, heat sesame oil over medium heat.
2. Add tempeh cubes and cook until browned on all sides, about 5 minutes.
3. Add broccoli florets and bell pepper slices.
4. Cook for another 5 minutes, or until vegetables are tender-crisp.
5. Stir in teriyaki sauce and cook for another minute.
6. Serve hot over cooked brown rice, garnished with sesame seeds.

GLUTEN FREE BREAD

Gluten-Free Multi-Seed Bread

Preparation Time: 15 minutes

Serves: 1

Calories: 200 **Carbs:** 20g **Protein:** 5g **Fat:** 10g **Fiber:** 5g **Sodium:** 100mg

Ingredients:

1 1/2 cups gluten-free flour blend

1/2 cup almond flour

1/2 cup ground flaxseed

1/4 cup chia seeds

1/4 cup sunflower seeds

1/4 cup pumpkin seeds

2 teaspoons baking powder

1 teaspoon baking soda

1/2 teaspoon salt

2 tablespoons maple syrup

2 tablespoons apple cider vinegar

1 1/2 cups non-dairy milk

1/4 cup olive oil

1/4 cup water

Method of Preparation:

1. Preheat the oven to 350°F (175°C) and line a loaf pan with parchment paper.
2. In a large bowl, combine the gluten-free flour blend, almond flour, ground flaxseed, chia seeds, sunflower seeds, pumpkin seeds, baking powder, baking soda, and salt.
3. In a separate bowl, whisk together the maple syrup, apple cider vinegar, non-dairy milk, olive oil, and water.
4. Pour the wet ingredients into the dry ingredients and stir until well combined.
5. Pour the batter into the prepared loaf pan and smooth the top.
6. Bake for 50-60 minutes, or until a toothpick inserted into the center comes out clean.
7. Allow the bread to cool in the pan for 10 minutes, then remove it from the pan and transfer it to a wire rack to cool completely before slicing.

Gluten-Free Artisan Bread

Preparation Time: 15 minutes

Serves: 1

Calories: 150 **Carbs:** 30g **Protein:** 2g **Fat:** 3g **Fiber:** 2g
Sodium: 100mg

Ingredients:

2 cups gluten-free flour blend

1 teaspoon xanthan gum

1 teaspoon salt

1 tablespoon sugar

2 1/4 teaspoons instant yeast

1 1/4 cups warm water

1 tablespoon olive oil

1 tablespoon apple cider vinegar

Method of Preparation:

1. Preheat the oven to 375°F (190°C) and line a baking
    sheet with parchment paper.

2. In a large bowl, whisk together the gluten-free flour blend, xanthan gum, salt, sugar, and instant yeast.

3. Add the warm water, olive oil, and apple cider vinegar to the dry ingredients and stir until well combined.

4. Cover the bowl with plastic wrap and let the dough rise in a warm place for 30 minutes.

5. Shape the dough into a round loaf and place it on the prepared baking sheet.

6. Using a sharp knife, make a few slashes in the top of the loaf.

7. Bake for 30-35 minutes, or until the bread is golden brown and sounds hollow when tapped on the bottom.

8. Allow the bread to cool on a wire rack before slicing.

Gluten-Free Peasant Bread

Preparation Time: 15 minutes

Serves: 1

Calories: 200 **Carbs:** 30g **Protein:** 3g **Fat:** 8g **Fiber:** 2g
Sodium: 100mg

Ingredients:

2 cups gluten-free flour blend

1 teaspoon baking soda

1 teaspoon salt

1 tablespoon sugar

1 1/4 cups non-dairy milk

1 tablespoon apple cider vinegar

1/4 cup olive oil

Method of Preparation:

1. Preheat the oven to 375°F (190°C) and grease a 9x5-inch loaf pan.
2. In a large bowl, whisk together the gluten-free flour blend, baking soda, salt, and sugar.
3. In a separate bowl, mix together the non-dairy milk, apple cider vinegar, and olive oil.
4. Pour the wet ingredients into the dry ingredients and stir until well combined.
5. Pour the batter into the prepared loaf pan and smooth the top.

6. Bake for 30-35 minutes, or until a toothpick inserted into the center comes out clean.

7. Allow the bread to cool in the pan for 10 minutes, then remove it from the pan and transfer it to a wire rack to cool completely before slicing.

No-Knead Gluten-Free Bread

Preparation Time: 5 minutes (plus resting time)

Serves: 1

Calories: 150 **Carbs:** 30g **Protein:** 2g **Fat:** 2g **Fiber:** 2g **Sodium:** 100mg

Ingredients:

3 cups gluten-free flour blend

1 teaspoon xanthan gum

1 teaspoon salt

1 teaspoon instant yeast

1 1/2 cups warm water

1 tablespoon apple cider vinegar

1 tablespoon olive oil

Method of Preparation:

1. In a large bowl, whisk together the gluten-free flour blend, xanthan gum, salt, and instant yeast.

2. Add the warm water, apple cider vinegar, and olive oil to the dry ingredients and stir until well combined.

3. Cover the bowl with plastic wrap and let the dough sit at room temperature for 12-18 hours, or until doubled in size.

4. Preheat the oven to 450°F (230°C) and place a Dutch oven or heavy-bottomed pot with a lid in the oven to heat up.

5. Carefully remove the hot pot from the oven and line it with parchment paper.

6. Scrape the dough into the hot pot and smooth the top with a wet spatula.

7. Cover the pot with the lid and bake for 30 minutes.

8. Remove the lid and bake for an additional 10-15 minutes, or until the bread is golden brown and sounds hollow when tapped on the bottom.

9. Allow the bread to cool in the pot for 10 minutes, then transfer it to a wire rack to cool completely before slicing.

Homemade Gluten-Free Bread

Preparation Time: 15 minutes (plus rising time)

Serves: 1

Calories: 200 **Carbs:** 30g **Protein:** 3g **Fat:** 8g **Fiber:** 2g
Sodium: 100mg

Ingredients:

2 cups gluten-free flour blend

1 teaspoon xanthan gum

1 teaspoon salt

1 tablespoon sugar

1 1/4 cups warm water

1 tablespoon apple cider vinegar

1/4 cup olive oil

1 tablespoon instant yeast

Method of Preparation:

1. Preheat the oven to 375°F (190°C) and grease a 9x5-inch loaf pan.

2. In a large bowl, whisk together the gluten-free flour blend, xanthan gum, salt, and sugar.

3. In a separate bowl, mix together the warm water, apple cider vinegar, olive oil, and instant yeast.

4. Pour the wet ingredients into the dry ingredients and stir until well combined.

5. Pour the batter into the prepared loaf pan and smooth the top.

6. Cover the pan with a clean kitchen towel and let the dough rise in a warm place for 30-45 minutes, or until doubled in size.

7. Bake for 30-35 minutes, or until the bread is golden brown and sounds hollow when tapped on the bottom.

8. Allow the bread to cool in the pan for 10 minutes, then remove it from the pan and transfer it to a wire rack to cool completely before slicing.

SOUPS AND STEWS

Mushroom Soup

Preparation Time: 10 minutes

Serves: 4

Calories: 150 **Carbs:** 10g **Protein:** 5g **Fat:** 10g **Fiber:** 3g

Sodium: 100mg

Ingredients:

1 tablespoon olive oil

1 onion, chopped

2 garlic cloves, minced

1-pound mushrooms, sliced

4 cups vegetable broth

1 teaspoon dried thyme

A pinch of salt and pepper

1/2 cup coconut cream (from a can)

Fresh parsley, for garnish

Method of Preparation:

1. In a large pot, heat olive oil over medium heat.
2. Add onion and garlic, and sauté until softened, about 5 minutes.

3. Add sliced mushrooms and cook until they release their juices, about 8-10 minutes.

4. Add vegetable broth, dried thyme, salt, and pepper. Bring to a simmer and cook for another 10 minutes.

5. Using an immersion blender, blend the soup until smooth. Alternatively, transfer the soup to a blender and blend until smooth, then return it to the pot.

6. Stir in coconut cream and cook for another 5 minutes.

7. Serve hot, garnished with fresh parsley.

Slow-Cooker Mediterranean Stew

Preparation Time: 10 minutes

Serves: 4

Calories: 200 **Carbs:** 30g **Protein:** 10g **Fat:** 5g **Fiber:** 8g **Sodium:** 100mg

Ingredients:

1 can (14 oz) diced tomatoes

1 can (14 oz) chickpeas, drained and rinsed

1 onion, chopped

2 garlic cloves, minced

1 bell pepper, chopped

1 zucchini, chopped

1/2 cup sliced black olives

1 teaspoon dried oregano

1 teaspoon dried basil

A pinch of salt and pepper

2 cups vegetable broth

Cooked quinoa or rice, for serving

Fresh parsley, for garnish

Method of Preparation:

1. In a slow cooker, combine diced tomatoes, chickpeas, onion, garlic, bell pepper, zucchini, black olives, dried oregano, dried basil, salt, and pepper.

2. Pour vegetable broth over the ingredients and stir to combine.

3. Cover and cook on low for 6-8 hours, or on high for 3-4 hours.

4. Serve hot over cooked quinoa or rice, garnished with fresh parsley.

Egg Drop Soup

Preparation Time: 5 minutes

Serves: 4

Calories: 100 **Carbs:** 5g **Protein:** 6g **Fat:** 5g **Fiber:** 1g
Sodium: 150mg

Ingredients:

4 cups vegetable broth

2 green onions, thinly sliced

1 tablespoon soy sauce

1 teaspoon sesame oil

A pinch of salt and pepper

Fresh cilantro, for garnish

Method of Preparation:

1. In a large pot, bring vegetable broth to a simmer over medium heat.
2. Add green onions, soy sauce, and sesame oil.
3. Stir to combine.

4. Cook for another minute, then season with salt and pepper.

5. Serve hot, garnished with fresh cilantro.

Special Cabbage Stew

Preparation Time: 10 minutes

Serves: 4

Calories: 150 **Carbs:** 20g **Protein:** 5g **Fat:** 5g **Fiber:** 8g **Sodium:** 90mg

Ingredients:

1 tablespoon olive oil

1 onion, chopped

2 carrots, chopped

2 celery stalks, chopped

1 small head cabbage, chopped

1 can (14 oz) diced tomatoes

4 cups vegetable broth

1 teaspoon dried thyme

A pinch of salt and pepper

Fresh parsley, for garnish

Method of Preparation:

1. In a large pot, heat olive oil over medium heat.
2. Add onion, carrots, and celery.
3. Sauté until vegetables are softened, about 5 minutes.
4. Add chopped cabbage and cook for another 5 minutes.
5. Stir in diced tomatoes, vegetable broth, dried thyme, salt, and pepper.
6. Bring to a simmer and cook for 20-30 minutes, or until the vegetables are tender.
7. Serve hot, garnished with fresh parsley.

Creamy Potato Leek Soup

Preparation Time: 15 minutes

Serves: 4

Calories: 250 **Carbs:** 30g **Protein:** 5g **Fat:** 10g **Fiber:** 5g **Sodium:** 100mg

Ingredients:

2 tablespoons olive oil

2 leeks, white and light green parts only, chopped

3 garlic cloves, minced

4 cups vegetable broth

4 cups diced potatoes

1 teaspoon dried thyme

A pinch of salt and pepper

1 cup coconut cream (from a can)

Fresh chives, for garnish

Method of Preparation:

1. In a large pot, heat olive oil over medium heat.
2. Add chopped leeks and garlic. Sauté until softened, about 5 minutes.
3. Add vegetable broth, diced potatoes, dried thyme, salt, and pepper.
4. Bring to a simmer and cook for 20-30 minutes, or until the potatoes are tender.

5. Using an immersion blender, blend the soup until smooth. Alternatively, transfer the soup to a blender and blend until smooth, then return it to the pot.

6. Stir in coconut cream and cook for another 5 minutes.

7. Serve hot, garnished with fresh chives.

Lentil Soup

Preparation Time: 10 minutes

Serves: 4

Calories: 200 **Carbs:** 30g **Protein:** 10g **Fat:** 5g **Fiber:** 10g **Sodium:** 100mg

Ingredients:

1 tablespoon olive oil

1 onion, chopped

2 carrots, chopped

2 celery stalks, chopped

2 garlic cloves, minced

1 cup dried lentils, rinsed

4 cups vegetable broth

1 can (14 oz) diced tomatoes

1 teaspoon dried thyme

A pinch of salt and pepper

Fresh parsley, for garnish

Method of Preparation:

1. In a large pot, heat olive oil over medium heat.
2. Add onion, carrots, celery, and garlic. Sauté until vegetables are softened, about 5 minutes.
3. Add dried lentils, vegetable broth, diced tomatoes, dried thyme, salt, and pepper.
4. Bring to a simmer and cook for 20-30 minutes, or until the lentils are tender.
5. Serve hot, garnished with fresh parsley.

DESSERTS

Lemon-Blueberry Poke Cake

Preparation Time: 15 minutes

Serves: 12

Calories: 350 **Carbs:** 45g **Protein:** 3g **Fat:** 18g **Fiber:** 1g **Sodium:** 100mg

Ingredients:

1 box gluten-free lemon cake mix

1 cup water

1/3 cup vegetable oil

1/2 cup lemon juice

1/2 cup blueberry jam

1 cup fresh blueberries

1 can (14 oz) sweetened condensed coconut milk

Method of Preparation:

1. Preheat the oven to 350°F (175°C) and grease a 9x13-inch baking dish.
2. In a large bowl, combine the gluten-free lemon cake mix, water, and vegetable oil.
3. Mix until well combined.
4. Pour the batter into the prepared baking dish and bake according to the package instructions.

5. While the cake is baking, combine lemon juice, blueberry jam, and sweetened condensed coconut milk in a saucepan over medium heat.

6. Cook until the mixture is smooth and well combined.

7. Remove the cake from the oven and use the handle of a wooden spoon to poke holes all over the top of the cake.

8. Pour the lemon-blueberry mixture over the cake, making sure it fills the holes.

9. Sprinkle fresh blueberries over the top of the cake.

10. Allow the cake to cool completely before serving.

Oatmeal Cookie Fruit Pizza

Preparation Time: 20 minutes

Serves: 8

Calories: 300 **Carbs:** 40g **Protein:** 3g **Fat:** 15g **Fiber:** 3g **Sodium:** 150mg

Ingredients:

1 1/2 cups gluten-free oats

1 cup gluten-free flour blend

1/2 teaspoon baking soda

1/2 teaspoon cinnamon

1/4 teaspoon salt

1/2 cup coconut oil, melted

1/2 cup maple syrup

1 teaspoon vanilla extract

8 oz dairy-free cream cheese

1/4 cup powdered sugar

Assorted fresh fruits (such as strawberries, kiwi, and blueberries), sliced

Method of Preparation:

1. Preheat the oven to 350°F (175°C) and line a baking sheet with parchment paper.
2. In a large bowl, combine oats, gluten-free flour blend, baking soda, cinnamon, and salt.
3. In a separate bowl, mix together melted coconut oil, maple syrup, and vanilla extract.
4. Pour the wet ingredients into the dry ingredients and stir until well combined.

5. Press the dough into a thin, round crust on the prepared baking sheet.

6. Bake for 12-15 minutes, or until golden brown. Allow to cool completely.

7. In a bowl, mix together dairy-free cream cheese and powdered sugar until smooth.

8. Spread the cream cheese mixture over the cooled cookie crust.

9. Arrange sliced fruits over the cream cheese layer.

10. Slice and serve.

Apple Crisp with Cranberries

Preparation Time: 15 minutes

Serves: 6

Calories: 250 **Carbs:** 35g **Protein:** 2g **Fat:** 12g **Fiber:** 5g **Sodium:** 10mg

Ingredients:

4 cups sliced apples

1/2 cup dried cranberries

1/4 cup maple syrup

1 teaspoon cinnamon

1/2 teaspoon nutmeg

1/2 cup gluten-free oats

1/4 cup gluten-free flour blend

1/4 cup coconut sugar

1/4 cup coconut oil, melted

1/4 cup chopped pecans

Method of Preparation:

1. Preheat the oven to 350°F (175°C) and grease a baking dish.
2. In a large bowl, combine sliced apples, dried cranberries, maple syrup, cinnamon, and nutmeg.
3. Mix until well combined.
4. Spread the apple mixture evenly in the prepared baking dish.
5. In a separate bowl, combine oats, gluten-free flour blend, coconut sugar, melted coconut oil, and chopped pecans. Mix until crumbly.

6. Sprinkle the oat mixture over the apples in the baking dish.

7. Bake for 30-35 minutes, or until the apples are tender and the topping is golden brown.

8. Serve warm.

Flaky Apple Pie Bars

Preparation Time: 20 minutes

Serves: 12 bars

Calories: 250 **Carbs:** 35g **Protein:** 2g **Fat:** 12g **Fiber:** 3g **Sodium:** 150mg

Ingredients:

2 cups gluten-free flour blend

1/2 teaspoon salt

1/2 cup cold unsalted butter, cubed

1/4 cup cold water

5 cups peeled and thinly sliced apples

1/2 cup sugar

2 tablespoons gluten-free flour blend

1 teaspoon ground cinnamon

1/4 teaspoon ground nutmeg

1/4 teaspoon ground allspice

1/4 teaspoon salt

Method of Preparation:

1. Preheat the oven to 350°F (175°C) and grease a 9x13-inch baking dish.
2. In a large bowl, combine 2 cups gluten-free flour blend and 1/2 teaspoon salt.
3. Cut in the cold butter until the mixture resembles coarse crumbs. Gradually add the cold water, tossing with a fork until the dough forms a ball.
4. Divide the dough in half.
5. Roll out half of the dough to fit the bottom of the prepared baking dish.
6. Place the dough in the dish and press it down evenly.
7. In a separate bowl, combine the sliced apples, sugar, 2 tablespoons gluten-free flour blend, cinnamon, nutmeg, allspice, and 1/4 teaspoon salt.
8. Mix until the apples are coated.

9. Spread the apple mixture evenly over the dough in the baking dish.

10. Roll out the remaining dough and place it over the apple mixture.

11. Press the edges to seal.

12. Bake for 45-50 minutes, or until the crust is golden brown.

13. Allow the bars to cool before slicing into squares.

Sweet Potato Bread Pudding with Pecan Praline Sauce

Preparation Time: 20 minutes

Serves: 8

Calories: 400 **Carbs:** 50g **Protein:** 6g **Fat:** 20g **Fiber:** 3g **Sodium:** 150mg

Ingredients:

4 cups gluten-free bread cubes

1 cup mashed sweet potatoes

1/2 cup sugar

1 teaspoon vanilla extract

1/2 teaspoon ground cinnamon

1/4 teaspoon ground nutmeg

1/4 teaspoon ground allspice

2 cups milk

1/2 cup chopped pecans

1/2 cup brown sugar

1/4 cup butter

1/4 cup heavy cream

Method of Preparation:

1. Preheat the oven to 350°F (175°C) and grease a 9x13-inch baking dish.
2. In a large bowl, combine the gluten-free bread cubes and mashed sweet potatoes.
3. In a separate bowl, whisk together the sugar, vanilla extract, cinnamon, nutmeg, allspice, and milk. Pour the mixture over the bread and sweet potatoes, stirring to combine.

4. Pour the bread pudding mixture into the prepared baking dish.

5. In a small saucepan, combine the chopped pecans, brown sugar, butter, and heavy cream. Cook over medium heat until the butter is melted and the sugar is dissolved.

6. Pour the pecan praline sauce over the bread pudding.

7. Bake for 40-45 minutes, or until the bread pudding is set and golden brown.

8. Serve warm, drizzled with additional pecan praline sauce if desired.

SALAD

Strawberry Spinach Salad with Avocado & Walnuts

Preparation Time: 10 minutes

Serves: 4

Calories: 250 **Carbs:** 15g **Protein:** 4g **Fat:** 20g **Fiber:** 6g
Sodium: 50mg

Ingredients:

4 cups baby spinach

1 cup sliced strawberries

1 avocado, diced

1/2 cup chopped walnuts

1/4 cup balsamic vinegar

2 tablespoons olive oil

1 tablespoon honey

A pinch of salt and pepper

Method of Preparation:

1. In a large bowl, combine baby spinach, sliced strawberries, diced avocado, and chopped walnuts.
2. In a small bowl, whisk together balsamic vinegar, olive oil, honey, salt, and pepper.
3. Pour the dressing over the salad and toss to combine.
4. Serve immediately.

Kale & Strawberry Salad

Preparation Time: 10 minutes

Serves: 4

Calories: 200 **Carbs:** 15g **Protein:** 6g **Fat:** 15g **Fiber:** 4g **Sodium:** 100mg

Ingredients:

4 cups chopped kale

1 cup sliced strawberries

1/4 cup sliced almonds

1/4 cup crumbled feta cheese

2 tablespoons balsamic vinegar

1 tablespoon olive oil

1 teaspoon honey

A pinch of salt and pepper

Method of Preparation:

1. In a large bowl, combine chopped kale, sliced strawberries, sliced almonds, and crumbled feta cheese.

2. In a small bowl, whisk together balsamic vinegar, olive oil, honey, salt, and pepper.

3. Pour the dressing over the salad and toss to combine.

4. Serve immediately.

Quinoa, Avocado & Chickpea Salad over Mixed Greens

Preparation Time: 15 minutes

Serves: 4

Calories: 300 **Carbs:** 30g **Protein:** 8g **Fat:** 15g **Fiber:** 10g **Sodium:** 100mg

Ingredients:

1 cup cooked quinoa

1 avocado, diced

1 can (14 oz) chickpeas, drained and rinsed

4 cups mixed greens

1/4 cup lemon juice

2 tablespoons olive oil

1 teaspoon Dijon mustard

A pinch of salt and pepper

Method of Preparation:

1. In a large bowl, combine cooked quinoa, diced avocado, and chickpeas.
2. In a small bowl, whisk together lemon juice, olive oil, Dijon mustard, salt, and pepper.
3. Pour the dressing over the quinoa mixture and toss to combine.
4. Serve over mixed greens.

Kale & Avocado Salad with Blueberries & Edamame

Preparation Time: 10 minutes

Serves: 4

Calories: 250 **Carbs:** 20g **Protein:** 8g **Fat:** 15g **Fiber:** 7g **Sodium:** 50mg

Ingredients:

4 cups chopped kale

1 avocado, diced

1/2 cup blueberries

1/2 cup shelled edamame

1/4 cup sliced almonds

2 tablespoons lemon juice

2 tablespoons olive oil

1 teaspoon honey

A pinch of salt and pepper

Method of Preparation:

1. In a large bowl, combine chopped kale, diced avocado, blueberries, shelled edamame, and sliced almonds.
2. In a small bowl, whisk together lemon juice, olive oil, honey, salt, and pepper.
3. Pour the dressing over the salad and toss to combine.
4. Serve immediately.

Grilled Caesar Salad

Preparation Time: 10 minutes

Serves: 2

Calories: 200 **Carbs:** 10g **Protein:** 5g **Fat:** 15g **Fiber:** 5g **Sodium:** 100mg

Ingredients:

1 head romaine lettuce, halved lengthwise

1 tablespoon olive oil

1/4 cup grated Parmesan cheese

1/4 cup gluten-free croutons

Caesar dressing (store-bought or homemade)

Method of Preparation:

1. Preheat a grill or grill pan over medium-high heat.
2. Brush the cut sides of the romaine lettuce with olive oil.
3. Place the lettuce on the grill cut side down and grill for 2-3 minutes, or until lightly charred.
4. Remove the lettuce from the grill and place it on a serving plate.
5. Drizzle with Caesar dressing, sprinkle with grated Parmesan cheese, and top with gluten-free croutons.
6. Serve immediately.

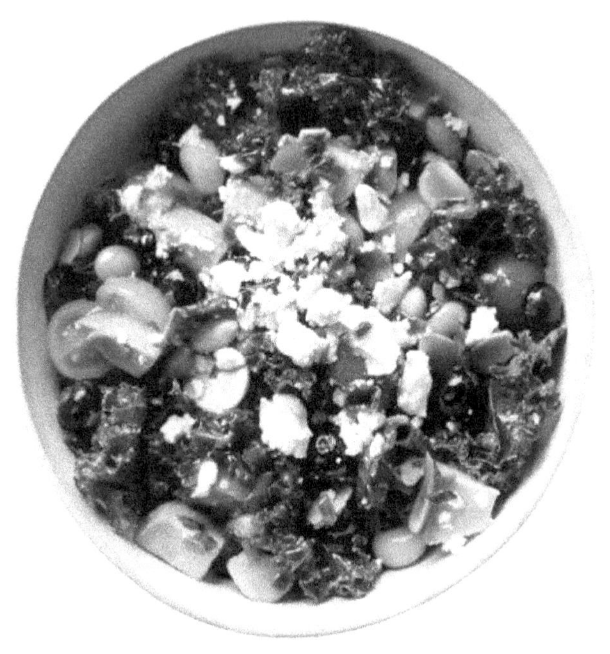

CONCLUSION

In conclusion, this book offers a diverse range of delicious and nutritious recipes that cater to you with dietary restrictions.

By focusing on plant-based ingredients, these recipes not only support a cruelty-free lifestyle but also provide numerous health benefits.

More so, this cookbook emphasizes the importance of incorporating anti-inflammatory foods into daily meals to reduce inflammation in the body, which can lead to various health issues if left unchecked.

The recipes are carefully crafted to include ingredients known for their anti-inflammatory properties, such as fruits, vegetables, whole grains, nuts, and seeds.

Each recipe is designed to be easy to prepare, making it accessible for home cooks of all skill levels.

Finally, by using simple and wholesome ingredients, the cookbook encourages you to embrace a healthier way of eating without sacrificing flavor or satisfaction.

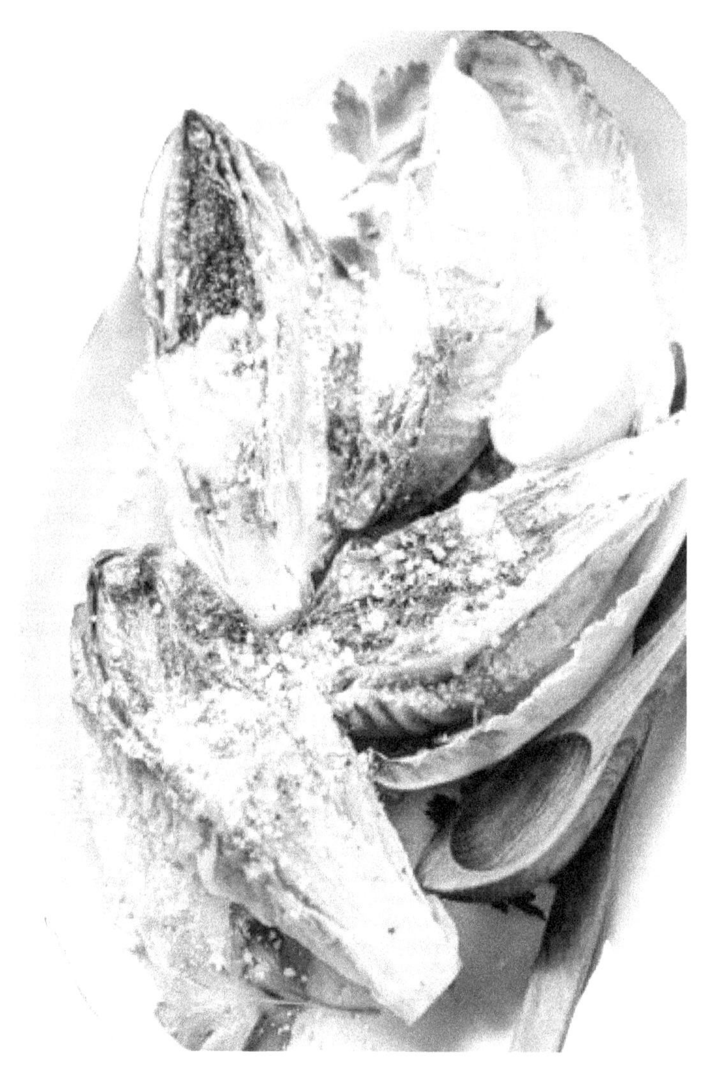